Table of

Introduction................................	
Ready-Made Meals & Snacks..	
Cauliflower Recipes – The Surprising Super Food.......................	Pg. 8
Main Dishes...	Pg. 12
Appetizers & Salads..	Pg. 20
Desserts & Other Treats...	Pg. 22
Acknowledgements...	Pg. 29

"A healthy outside starts from the inside." -Robert Urich

INTRODUCTION

My purpose for sharing my life story is simple. I want to help others who find themselves in a situation similar to mine. I want to show you how I was able to conquer the twin challenges of diabetes and weight control, in the hope that others may find the inspiration to do the same.

The 2015 Canadian Diabetes Association website states that "over 9 million Canadians are living with diabetes or prediabetes. Chances are diabetes affects you or someone you know." That means one in every four Canadians is facing some difficult decisions about their health, weight, food choices and lifestyle.

Although diet is only one instrument in the toolbox to fight diabetes, our complex relationship with food makes it one of the most important factors involved in determining our success or failure at managing our condition. And for a foodie like me, it became my ultimate challenge.

By finding ways to enjoy my food, without feeling deprived or restricted, and embracing the need for regular physical activity, I was able to accomplish something I never thought possible. I was able to create a new, healthier lifestyle and a fresh, confident, optimistic outlook for the future.

This is what I wish for you.

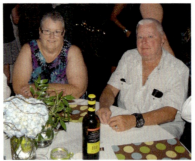

At the beginning of my health &
weight loss journey
With my husband, Larry
August, 2011

From Dictionary.com: FOODIE (foo-dee),
- (noun, slang)
- a person keenly interested in food, especially in eating or cooking

That's me. I am a foodie. I love preparing and eating delicious food. It has been my pride and joy in happy times, my solace and comfort in tough times. Simply put, food has played a very important part in my life. For many years, though, my attitudes towards food have had a negative impact on my health.

But not anymore.

I'm writing this to tell you my story in the hope that you can apply some of the things I have learned to your own life living with diabetes and dealing with the issues surrounding food and lifestyle. This is a story about facing our own reality, making a decision to do something about it, and actively educating ourselves in order to have the correct information to make better choices.

My journey towards a healthier lifestyle has taken me to places I never dreamed I could be. I look better, feel better, can do things and go places that were simply just wishful thinking before. I want you to know that improving our lives is doable. It's never too late to start. Food can become our friend, not our enemy. I know because I did it and now I enjoy my life.

And if I can do it, you can too.

MY STORY

I was born Ruth Elaine Charters in Hamilton, Ontario, on January 1, 1947. From a child, I always loved my food, but never had a significant weight issue growing up. We had a normal family life -- my dad worked at Westinghouse and, like most families, my mom stayed at home and looked after the family. A little brother came along rather late in my parents' lives, and at age 11, I became the big sister to a baby that I often mothered as if he were my own.

In high school, I enjoyed a few close friends, and life was pretty normal. It wasn't until I met my high school sweetheart, Larry Charles Lynn Pepper, and married him on August 27, 1966, that things began to change. I started to gain weight. By the time our two daughters were born, one in 1969 and one in 1972, a pattern of creeping weight gain had been established. Food became a struggle. I knew that if I ate this or that the scales would silently condemn me and, in my mind, there was no way I could win this battle. From time to time, I tried calorie restrictive diets, lost and gained again, and felt deprived and unhappy until I simply gave up.

By the age of 64, I was struggling with the cumulative effects of high cholesterol, high blood pressure, depression, and finally Type 2 diabetes. I was more than 100 pounds overweight. I couldn't walk very far, and certainly not around the block. I leaned on shopping carts in stores to relieve the excruciating pain in my hips and feet. I broke my foot twice when I slipped on ice and landed with the full force of my weight on my foot. I was wearing a 5X plus size top and facing the prospect of paying outrageous prices for specialty clothes that would fit me. My self-esteem was in the dumper and my spirits were low.

I was on five different kinds of medications for all my conditions, but it was the diabetes medication that finally did me in. I suffered a severe side effect from it, becoming very sick and feeling decidedly rotten. The doctor took me off it and did not prescribe anything else until the drug was completely out of my system.

Oprah would have called it "an Ah-Ha moment."

I knew I was in serious trouble if I did nothing, and there was only one thing I could do -- lose the weight that was dragging me down, both physically and mentally. I had no choice. It was either do it or die.

My first visit to the Diabetic Clinic at Norfolk General Hospital, in Simcoe, Ontario, was an amazing accomplishment for me, simply because I was confronting the reality of my situation and doing something about it. However, it was the competent, professional staff there who literally saved the day for me. For the first time in my life, I was paired with a dietitian who was truly inspiring. She did not talk down to me, nor did she make me feel ashamed or inferior. She gave me a very simple diet, in an easy-to-read format, customized especially for me. On a human level, we bonded instantly and I began to see one tiny pinprick of light at the end of a very long, dark tunnel.

I was on my way to a new me, and I couldn't be more excited.

Basically, I could consume 45 carbs per meal at three meals per day, with one 15-carb snack per day. I learned how to check food labels for carbohydrate and fibre values and to choose foods appropriate to controlling blood sugar levels. A nurse checked my feet and blood pressure and taught me how to monitor my sugar levels. At the Diabetic Foot Clinic, I was monitored on a regular basis. My feet were examined, tested for feeling, and toe nails trimmed. The support system offered by these professionals was absolutely outstanding. Most surprising was the fact that this service is provided absolutely free to the patient.

With all this help, I began to lose about four to eight pounds a month. As time went on, and the weight came off, two to four pounds per month became the norm.

To date I have lost a total of 90 pounds and gained my life back -- and a happy, enjoyable one to boot. At the age of 68, I have more energy than I would ever have thought possible. I can walk all over the Town of Simcoe. I eat delicious foods, make fabulous dishes, and never feel deprived of anything. My blood sugar levels have been consistently within acceptable ranges. I can now shop off the rack at many regular clothing shops. I can volunteer, join clubs, exercise and meet new people with poise and confidence. I have this amazing support system at the clinic and among a close circle of friends. Best of all, when I look in the mirror, I see the new me. I'm happier and more optimistic than I have ever been. My eyes sparkle again, my skin glows again, I've gained my shape back and actually notice some muscle definition. Even my dentist said my gums and dental health has improved enormously.

Remarkably, and perhaps best of all, my attitude towards food has changed. I still love food, and I still love preparing and eating it. I still have unhealthy cravings but I have learned how to satisfy them in a healthy way. The bottom line is, I no longer consider my new way of eating as a diabetic diet, but rather as a whole new way of life.

What I really would like people to know is, this is not impossible. If I can do it, you can too.

Follow me as I explain in more detail some of the tips and hints that can make you successful in your quest for better health.

The Value of Exercise

One of the most valuable pieces of advice you will get is about the importance of exercise in maintaining blood sugar levels and controlling weight. We all have certain entrenched attitudes towards exercise, and commonly, many people avoid it. I want to stress that without committing myself to regular physical activity, I would not have been as successful at attaining my health goal. In fact, without the benefits of regular exercise, I may not have gotten the results I wanted, and once again, I may have given up.

I started out on a recumbent stationary bike and I joined a water aerobics class. Both of these activities were much gentler on the joints in the hips, knees and ankles than other options. The recumbent bike is outfitted with a chair instead of a saddle, so it is much more comfortable than conventional stationary bikes. Your torso is in an upright position, your feet are out in front of you and your whole body feels less stressed. I could put a pillow on the seat for more cushioning, and listen to my favourite music while I exercised. Weather, of course, was never a factor and, in the beginning, I loved the privacy of my home.

Once I started seeing some results on the bike, I decided to try walking around the block. Gradually, I was able to cover more distance, increasing my walks to two blocks, then three. Today I can walk anywhere in the Town of Simcoe. My feet have become my preferred mode of transportation, and I will choose to walk more times than I will choose to drive. (Just think of the gas you will save!) I take advantage of all the beautiful trails and miles of pedestrian sidewalks that we are so lucky to have. The fresh air and scenery is invigorating and I meet dozens of lovely people along the way.

Eventually, I began to notice a co-relation between when I ate and when I exercised and the effect that the timing of those two activities had on my blood sugar levels. If my sugar levels were a little high, I would exercise to bring them down. I could tell that I got a maximum benefit from scheduling my food intake and exercise periods in this way.

The Art of Reading Labels

In Canada, we are very lucky to be provided with the nutritional analysis of most foods we purchase. Reading labels is key to understanding exactly what we are putting in our mouths, and for us diabetics, it is critical.

Because of the simplicity of the meal plan chart provided by my dietitian, I found the carbohydrate, calorie and fibre values on food labels was not confusing. In fact, I began to make it a game to find the foods I loved with the least carb values but the maximum serving size. That way, I never felt deprived of anything, and always felt I was able to eat reasonable amounts without going over my carb limit. I do want to caution you, however, that some low-carb foods are actually higher in calories than others. This might sabotage your efforts to lose weight, so you must be careful about the foods you choose.

What Worked For Me Could Work For You

Let's face it, anyone can roast some chicken and steam some vegetables, but it's a bit harder to find other ready-made products that fit the carb/calorie diet plan. I probably spent unreasonable amounts of time reading labels in grocery stores, but eventually it paid off. I was able to make a workable list of products that not only taste delicious, but kept me within acceptable carb and calorie ranges. The following are a few of my favourites:

1. Meats and Main Dishes:

Marc Angelo Mild Italian Style Turkey Burgers
Marc Angelo Turkey Sausages (both available at Food Basics)

I love burgers and sausages, and these are delicious. The burgers have 150 calories and 3 carbs. The sausages have 30 calories and 1 carb. To jazz up the burgers a bit, I sprinkle them with Garlic and Herb Clubhouse seasoning (which contains no salt) before cooking.

McCain's Ultra Thin Crust Pizza (available at most grocery stores)

A good alternative when you are short on time. Pair it with a nutritious salad and supper is ready. A quarter of a pizza contains 13 carbs.

2. Snacks and Desserts:

I looked extensively for snacks and dessert items under 15 carbs and these are my favourites (available in most grocery stores):

Fibre One Bars
Delights Lemon - 13 carbs
Chocolate Chip - 13 carbs
Peanut Butter - 13 carbs
Caramel Nut - 12 carbs
Brownies - 12 carbs

Snack Pack Pudding (no sugar added)
Vanilla - 8 carbs
Chocolate - 8 carbs

Apple Sauce Snacks - (unsweetened)
8 carbs each

Nature Valley Granola Thins
Peanut Butter Flavour - 3 carbs

Irresistibles Brand Frozen Yogurt Bars - available at Food Basics
3 flavours - 9 carbs each

Because I enjoy my snacks so much, I compiled a list of products which tasted good and gave me a maximum serving size with the least amount of carbs. The following products fall into the "chips and cheezies" category, and by choosing them, I get a low carb value without feeling deprived of my favourite kind of snack.

Pepperidge Farms Cracker Chips: (come in a variety of flavours and available at most grocery stores)
Nacho   16 crackers = 14 carbs
Ketchup   20 crackers = 14 carbs
MultiGrain   20 crackers = 14 carbs
Barbecue   20 crackers = 15 carbs
Chocolate   20 crackers = 14 carbs
Creamy Caramel   20 crackers = 14 carbs

Breton Crackers - Popped
ChickpeaRed Bean Chili   14 crackers = 12 carbs
Chickpea Sea Salt and Pepper   14 crackers = 12 carbs

Special K Brand Crackers
Sour Cream & Onion   17 crackers = 12 carbs

Chee Cha Puffs- various flavours (available at Wal-Mart and Bulk Barn stores)
2 cups = 16 carbs

Skinny Sticks
13 sticks = 14 carbs

3. Salad Dressings:

Salad dressings are a little trickier because some salad dressings are low carb but high calories. I learned that the hard way when I stopped losing weight, and began to gain one or two pounds very slowly over time, due in part to high calorie salad dressings.

This is what I recommend:

Irresistibles Smart Life Brand (available at Food Basics):
Sundried Tomato and Oregano - 1 teaspoon = 3 carbs, 15 calories
Tzatziki Greek Yogurt - 1 teaspoon = 1 carb, 30 calories
Honey Dijon - 1 teaspoon = 3 carbs, 15 calories

4. Toppings and Spices:

Club House Salad Toppings - great to add to salads for extra crunch
1 tbsp = 30 calories, 2 carbs

Club House Salad Herbs - add these to salads for extra flavour
1/2 tsp = 0 calories, 1 carb

Club House Parmesan & Herbs - a wonderful product to sprinkle on popcorn, or on vegetables or meat while cooking
1/2 tsp = 0 calories, 0 carbs

Club House Garlic & Herbs - adds zip to cooked vegetables and meat
1/4 tsp = 0 calories, 1 carb

RECIPES

Even if you're not keen about cooking, I encourage you to experiment with low carb recipes simply because some are so simple and so delicious you will be astounded. After all, a good meal is a very satisfying thing, and if it's easy, tasty, low carb and low calorie, what's not to like? Enjoying our food, while staying within healthy carb and calorie limits, makes us feel less deprived and more likely to embrace our new way of eating as a new way of life.

The on-line world is a treasure trove of fantastic recipes and I encourage you to check out websites like "Pinterest" or Google "low carb recipes". However, not all recipes will provide a carb and calorie count. If you have an interesting recipe, or perhaps one passed down by generations in your family, the Diabetic Clinic will calculate the carb and calorie values, and show you how to alter the recipe to bring those values in line with your daily limits. Remember, the dietitians and professional staff are there to help you, and many times I have turned to them for assistance in this respect.

The most practical thing I learned was to freeze meat dishes, casseroles, soups and chilis in one person servings. That way, not only do you have a quick and tasty meal ready when it's time to eat, but you eliminate the temptation to just "grab whatever" when meal time rolls around. This is also a helpful tip when others in your family insist on eating whatever they like, rather than taking into consideration what's best for you.

Cauliflower: The Super Food That is Most Surprising!

I've discovered cauliflower is a most versatile vegetable. With a little imagination, we can make it taste like potato salad or like fried rice! Never again show up at a barbecue feeling like you can't enjoy the inevitable bowl of potato salad because of your diabetes!

Here's my version of **Mock Potato Salad**:

Use the ingredients you would use to make your own potato salad, but substitute cauliflower for the potatoes! **Important tip:** just steam the cauliflower until it's still a little crunchy, then put it in ice water to stop it from cooking further. Drain it well, and put it in the refrigerator to cool completely. Make sure you re-drain it once more. (You don't want it to turn out runny.)

Add onions, celery, hard-boiled eggs and pepper. Toss it with Miracle Whip, a bit of mustard and some sweetner to taste.

The end result? A carb-free dish you can't tell from real potato salad. How hard is that?

Read on for more delicious cauliflower recipes.

Carb-Free Cauliflower Fried Rice: (I found this one on Pinterest)
(from Family Fresh Meals at http://www.familyfreshmeals.com)

Ingredients:
3 cups of raw grated cauliflower (use a cheese grater or food processor)
1/2 cup frozen peas
1/2 cup carrots, thinly sliced
3-4 cloves garlic, minced
1/2 cup diced onion
1/2 tablespoon olive oil
2 eggs (or 4 egg whites scrambled)
3 tablespoons soy sauce

Instructions:
1. In a large pan, saute garlic and onions in olive oil on a medium/high heat, until onions become soft and transparent (about 2-3 minutes).

2. Add peas and carrots. Cook until carrots begin to soften and peas are heated through (about 3-4 minutes).

3. Stir in scrambled eggs, cauliflower and soy sauce. Cook stirring frequently about 5-7 minutes.

4. Add in your favourite protein and vegetable (I use mushrooms, broccoli and sometimes diced chicken).

Broccoli and Cauliflower Salad:
(from kraftcanada.com)

This is delicious -- a dish I serve company and take to potlucks.

Ingredients:
1 medium head of cauliflower, cut into florets, blanched
1 medium bunch of broccoli, cut into florets, blanched
1 medium onion, finely chopped
1 cup grated old cheddar cheese
1/2 cup of real bacon bits
1 cup Miracle Whip Original Spread
1 tsp mustard

Instructions:
Toss cauliflower, broccoli, onion, cheese and bacon bits in a large salad bowl. Mix Miracle Whip and mustard. Pour over salad, toss to coat. Cover and refrigerate.

(Blanching tip: To blanch vegetables, plunge into boiling water briefly (2 minutes), then into cold water to stop the cooking process. This will also retain the colour and flavour.)

Serving Size: 1/2 cup = 100 calories, 6 g. carbs, 2 g. fibre.

Low Carb Bacon-Cheddar Cauliflower Chowder
(from iowagirleats.com)

This excellent hearty soup is thick and cheesy and serves 8 people. Only 7 carbs per serving.

Ingredients:

8 slices bacon, chopped (half used for garnish)
1/2 small onion, chopped OR 1 tsp onion powder
1 celery stalk, chopped
2 garlic cloves, minced
salt & pepper
4 cups shredded or grated cauliflower (1/2 large head)
2 tbsp water
2 tbsp flour
2 cups chicken broth, divided
2 cups 2% milk
3-4 dashes hot sauce (or to taste)
2 1/2 cups shredded sharp cheddar cheese, divided (use half for garnish)
2 green onions, chopped (optional)

Instructions:

1. Whisk together flour and 1/2 cup chicken broth in small bowl, then set aside.
2. Saute bacon in large soup pot over medium heat until crisp. Using a slotted spoon, transfer bacon to a paper towel-lined plate, then remove all but 1 tbsp drippings from the pot. Add chopped onion, celery and garlic to the pot, then season with salt and pepper and saute until vegetables are tender, about 4-5 minutes.
3. Add cauliflower and onion powder (if using) to the pot, stir to combine. Add water then place a lid on top and steam cauliflower until tender, stirring a couple of times, about 5-7 minutes. Add remaining chicken broth and milk then turn up heat and bring to a boil.
4. Slowly whisk in flour/chicken broth mixture while stirring, then turn down heat and simmer for 3-4 minutes, or until chowder has thickened. Turn off heat, then stire in 2 cups cheddar cheese until smooth. Stir in half the cooked bacon. Taste and adjust salt, pepper and hot sauce if necessary. Serve topped with remaining cheddar cheese, cooked bacon and green onions.

"Let food be thy medicine and medicine be thy food" -Hippocrates

Carb Free Skinny Baked Cauliflower Tots:
(from brunchtimebaker.com)

These are fabulous, and so easy to prepare. Recipe makes about 20 tots.

Ingredients:

2 cups cauliflower florets
1 large egg
1/2 cup onion, minced
1/4 cup bell pepper, minced (optional)
1/2 cheddar cheese, shredded
1/4 parmesan Cheese
1/4 cup bread crumbs
1/4 cup minced cilantro or parsley (optional) (OR seasoning of your choice, I use Italian)
salt & pepper to taste
cooking spray or oil

Instructions:

1. Preheat oven to 375F. Spray nonstick cookie sheet with cooking spray or lightly grease with oil. Set aside. Steam cauliflower in hot water for 3-5 minutes or until nice and soft, drain and chop with knife or blend in food processor (just a few seconds).
2. In medium bowl, cmbine all of the ingredients and season with salt and pepper to taste.
3. Spoon about 1 tbsp of mixture in your hands and roll into small oval shaped tots.
4. Place on cookie sheet 1/2 inch apart and bake for about 20 minutes, trning halfway through cooking until golden.

Mashed Cauliflower
(from Company's Coming Low-Carb by Jean Pare)

Ingredients:

6 cups cauliflower florets
water
1/3 cup grated Parmesan cheese
1/4 cup light sour cream
2 tbsp butter or margarine softened
1/4 teasp salt

Instructions:

1. Cook cauliflower in waer in large saucepan on medium until tender. Drain. Mash.
2. Add remaining 5 ingredients. Mix until margarine is melted. Serves 6.

1 serving = 97 calories, 6 g. carbs, 2 g. fibre

Loaded Cauli & Buffalo Chicken Casserole:
(from loveandprimal.com)

If you want to impress your company with a dish "to die for", try this! My friends love it!

Ingredients:

2 lbs boneless, skinless chicken breasts, cut into 1/2 inch cubs
1 large cauliflower (florets)
1/3 cup olive oil
1 1/2 tsp salt
1 tbsp freshly ground pepper
1 tbsp paprika
2 tbsp garlic powder
6 tbsp hot sauce or buffalo sauce (I use less)

Topping:
2 cups Fiesta Blend ccheese or a mix of cheddar and Monterey Jack
1 cup cumbled bacon
1 cup diced green onion

Instructions:

1. Preheat oven to 400 F. In a large bowl mix together the olive oil, salt, pepper, paprika, garlic powder and hot sauce.
2. Add the cauliflower florets and stir to coat.
3. Scoop the cauliflower into a cooking spray coated 9x13 inch baking dish, leaving behind as much of the olive oil/hot sauce mix as possible.
4. Bake the cauliflower for 30-35 minutes, stirring every 10-15 minutes, until cooked through and starting to brown.
5. While the cauliflower is cooking, add the cubed chicken to the bowl with the leftover olive oil/hot sauce mix and stir to coat.
6. Once the cauliflower is fully cooked, remove from the oven.
7. Top the cooked cauliflower with the raw, marinated chicken.
8. In a bowl, mix together the cheese, bacon & green onion, and top the raw chicken with the cheese mix.
9. Return the casserole to the oven and bake for 15 minutes or until the chicken is cooked through and the topping is bubby delicious.
10. Drizzle with ranch dressing or blue cheese.
11. Serve with extra hot sauce and/or ranch dressing

Serves 6. One serving = 282 calories

MAIN DISHES

Tuna Cakes:
(By Vered DeLeeuw, healthyrecipesblogs.com)

Awesome entree! So tasty and delicious! Recipe can be halved very easily. You can make them, freeze them, then cook them at a later date too! I add 1/2 teaspoon of Club House Parmesan and Herb seasoning for added flavour.

Ingredients:

2 (4 oz.) cans tuna in water, well drained
1/2 cup quick-cooking oats
2 large eggs, lightly beaten
1/2 cup plain low fat Greek yogurt
1/2 teasp salt
1/4 teasp black pepper
1/2 cup choppedfreshparsley
2 tbsp olive oil for frying

Instructions:

1. In a medium bowl, use a fork to mix together the tuna, oats, eggs, yogurt, salt, pepper and parsley.
2. Heat the olive oil in a large nonstick skillet over medium heat, about 4 minutes.
3. Measuring 1/4 cup mixture for each cake, fry the tuna cakes 2-3 minuteson each side until golden brown. Serve immediately. Makes 8 cakes.

Serving size: 1 tuna cake = 111 calories, 4 g. carbs, 0 g. fibre

Ruth's Delicious Chili:

This is my own recipe, and I think you'll love it! Fill containers with single serving and freeze.

Ingredients:

1 lb ground beef (turkey or chicken)
1 pkg onion soup mix
1 large can kidney beans
1 can brown beans
1 can tomato soup
1 can stewed tomatoes
chili powder, salt & pepper to suit.

1. Brown the ground meat with onion soup mix.
2. Put this mixture in a large pot. Add remaining ingredients and simmer.

1 serving = 1 cup = 15 carbs

Cabbage Rolls:

This one is mine too, and it's a winner! I freeze two rolls for an individual serving size.

Ingredients:
One medium cabbage
2 lbs ground beef, or 1 lb ground beef and 1 lb ground pork
2 eggs
3 cups cooked rice
1 pkg onion soup mix
1 small tin tomato paste

Sauce:
4 tbsp brown sugar
1 cup chopped onion
2 cans tomato soup
1 large can tomato juice
4 bay leaves
8 whole cloves

Instructions:

1. Combine meat, eggs, rice, onion soup mix and tomato paste. Roll into cabbage leaves.
2. Place in roasting pan. Pour sauce over rolls.
3. Bake at 350F for two to three hours or until cabbage is soft.

1 cabbage roll = 15 carbs

SLOW COOKER POT ROAST:
(from kraftcanada.com)

Talk about comfort food! This is the ultimate! A breeze to make.

Ingredients:

1/2 cup Bull's Eye Bold Original barbecue sauce
1/2 cup water
1 pkg onion soup mix
1 boneless beef pot roast (2 1/2 lbs or 1.1 kg.)
1 lb. new red potatoes
1 pkg baby carrots
1 onion, thickly sliced

Instructions:

1. Mix first three ingredients.
2. Place meat in slow cooker. Top with vegetables and sauce. Cover.
3. Cook on low 8-9 hours, or on high 6 to 7 hours (depending on appliance).

Serving size: 1/10th recipe = 220 calories, 20 g. carbs, 2 g. fibre

Beef-Crusted Pizza:
(from Company's Coming Low-Carb by Jean Pare)

I tried this one on my friends and they raved about it. It's excellent! Try different toppings!

Ingredients:

1 1/2 lbs lean ground beef or ground chicken
1/3 cup grated part-skim mozzarella cheese
2 large eggs, fork beaten
2 tsp dried basil
1 tsp dried whole oregano
1 tsp pepper
1/2 tsp dried thyme

1/3 cup tomato sauce
2/3 cup grated part-skim mozzarella cheese
1 medium tomato sliced
4 1/2 oz can of sliced olives, drained
1/2 cup chopped green pepper

2/3 cup of Monterey Jack With Jalapeno cheese

Instructions:

1. Scramble fry ground beef in large non-stick fry pan on medium-high for 5 to 10 minutes until no longer pink. Drain. Transfer beef to large bowl. Cool.
2. Add next 7 ingredients. Stir well. Press beef mixture in bottom and halfway up side of greased 12 inch deep dish pizza pan. Bake in 400F oven for about 5 minutes until firm and cheese is melted. Let standfor 10 minutes.
3. Spoon tomato sauce onto beef crust. Spread evenly. Sprinkl second amount of mozzarella cheese over sauce. Layer next 3 ingredients, in order given, over cheese
4. Sprinkle with Monterey Jack cheese. Bake for 15 to 20 minutes until cheese is melted and golden. Cut into 6 wedges.

Serving size = 1 wedge = 341 calories, 8 g. carbs, 1 g. fibre.

BEEF AND CHICKEN POT PIES:

This is my own recipe. I make them in 4 inch foil tart shells and freeze them individually for a quick and easy supper for one. The trick to lowering the carb content is to only use a top crust!

Ingredients for beef:

900 grams lean ground beef
2 pkgs onion soup mix
1 pepper, chopped (yellow, red or orange are sweeter than green)
1/2 cup peas or vegetables of your choice
1 small pouch gravy mix
1 tbsp worcestershire sauce

Ingredients for chicken:

800 grams chopped cooked chicken
1/2 chopped pepper
1 medium potato, cubed (or use cauliflower to reduce carbs)
1/2 cup peas or vegetables of your choice
1 can chicken broth
2 cans creamed soup (chicken or mushroom)
seasoning to taste (I use pepper, garlic powder, and McCormick's No Salt Added Seasoned Herb Mix Medley

Instructions:

1. Brown the beef, if using beef.
2. Mix ingredients together and simmer for about 15 minutes.
3. Put mix into tart shells.
4. Top with crust and bake at 400F until crust is brown.

Makes 7 to 8 pies = 10 carbs each

SHEPHERD'S PIES:

This is also my own concoction, and I'm so sure you'll love it that you can call me up and complain if you don't!!

Use the same ingredients as for Beef or Chicken Pot Pies. Substitute mashed cauliflower for potatoes. (The mashed cauliflower lowers the carb value and tastes just as good!)

Put meat mixture in tart shell and top with mashed cauliflower and grated cheese. Bake as above.

HAMBURGER SOUP:
(from Pinterest, faithfulnessfarmblogrecipes)

If you want a hearty, satisfying soup, try this! A breeze to make and freezes well. Easy to microwave if you freeze individual servings!

Ingredients:

1 pound ground beef
4 stalks celery, coarsely chopped
1/2 cup onion, chopped
1 clove garlic, minced
1/2 medium (or 4 cups) cabbage, chopped
2 oz. fresh spinach, thinly sliced
2 cans beef broth
4 broth cans of water
8 oz. can of tomato sauce
2 tsp salt
1/2 tsp pepper

Instructions:

1. Brown hamburger with onion and celery. Drain fat.
2. Add cabbage, cook and stir until tender
3. Add all remaining ingredients, bring to boil.
4. Cover and simmer on low for about 2 hours. Adjust seasoning to taste.

Makes 8 servings. 1 serving = 126 calories, 5g. carbs, 2g fibre.

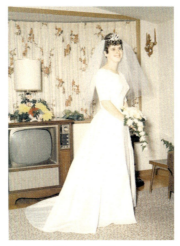

On my wedding day
August 27, 1966

STUFFED PEPPERS
(from Company's Coming Low-Carb, by Jean Pare)

Jean Pare is right when she says, "Chili-spiced beef fills tasty bell pepper halves. Melted cheese toping adds extra goodness!"

Ingredients:

3 large peppers, halved lengthwise, seeds and ribs removed
boiling water to cover
ice water

1 lb lean ground beef
1 cup medium salsa
1 1/2 tsp chili powder
1/2 cup grated light medium cheddar cheese
1/2 cup grated Monterey Jack cheese

Instructions:

1. Cook pepper halves in boiling water in medium saucepan for about 3 minutes until brightly coloured. Drain. Immediately plunge into ice water in medium bowl. Let stand for about 10 minutes until cold. Drain. Arrange pepper halves, skin-side down, in single layer in ungreased 3 quart (3L) shallow baking dish.
2. Scramble-fry ground beef in large non-stick frying pan on medium-high for 5 to 10 minutes until no longer pink. Remove from heat. Drain.
3. Add salsa and chili powder. Stir well. Divide and spoon beef mixture into each pepper half. Pack lightly.
4. Combine both cheeses in small bowl. Divide and sprinkle over top of beef mixture. Cook uncovered in 350F oven for 20 to 25 minutes until heated through and cheese is melted.

Makes 6 servings. 1 serving (one half pepper) = 222 calories, 9 g. carbs, 2 g. fibre.

"Take care of your body. It's the only place you have to live." -Jim Rohn

Hearty Ham Quiche:
(from Company's Coming Low-Carb, by Jean Pare)

This is a hearty ham quiche that will become your favourite. Substitute different meat and veggies, or any cheese, that tickles you! You can also use glutin-free cornstarch instead of flour. Freezes great in 3 inch tart shells for individual servings.

Ingredients:

2 tsp hard margarine, or butter
1 cup finely diced cooked ham
1 cup finely chopped cauliflower
1 cup sliced fresh white mushrooms

6 large eggs
3/4 cup milk
1 tbsp all-purpose flour
1/8 tsp salt
1/2 tsp pepper

3/4 cup grated Swiss Cheese

Instructions:

1. Melt margarine in large frying pan on medium. Add next 3 ingredients. Cook for 5 to 10 minutes, stirring occasionally, until cauliflower is tender-crisp and mushrooms are starting to brown. Transfer to medium bowl. Cool.
2. Beat next 5 ingredients with whisk in large bowl until smooth. Add ham mixture. Stir well. Pour into greased 9 inch pie plate.
3. Sprinkle with cheese. Bake in 350F oven for about 40 minutes until knife inserted in centre comes out clean. Let stand for 10 minutes. Cut into 6 wedges.

Serves 3. 1 serving = 420 calories, 10g carbs, 1 g. fibre.

LOW CALORIE PARMESAN CHICKEN
(from thinkingoutsidethepot.com)

You will be amazed at how simple and tasty this recipe is. My friends agreed it was so delicious, and it was no trouble at all to make.

Ingredients:

3 boneless, skinless chicken breasts
1/4 Parmesan cheese, grated
2 tbsp dried Italian bread crumbs
1/8 tsp paprika
1 tsp dried parsley
1/2 tsp garlic powder
1/4 tsp pepper
1 large Ziploc bag

Instructions:

1. Thaw chicken breast. Combine the rest of the ingredients in the Ziploc bag.
2. Preheat oven to 400F. Rinse chicken under warm water.
3. Place chicken in Ziploc bag and make sure each breast is covered completely.
4. Place in non-stick baking pan and bake for 30 minutes until chicken is no longer pink.

1 serving = 178 calories, 2 carbs

"You are never too old to set another goal or dream a new dream." -C.S. Lewis

APPETIZERS AND SALADS

Here are a couple of my favourite recipes that are great for barbecues, picnics and parties.

Bite-Size Bacon Spinach Cheese Balls:
(from sugardishme.com)

My granddaughter thinks this is the best! It's delicious, and it's carb-free!!

Ingredients:

5 slices bacon
5 oz. fresh spinach
1/2 tsp salt
1/2 cup onion, finely minced
2 cloves garlic, finely minced
1 (8 oz.) block of cream cheese, softened
1/2 cup shredded cheddar jack cheese
1/4 tsp cayenne pepper
1/2 cup walnuts or pecans, finely chopped

Instructions:

1. In large skillet, cook the bacon until crispy. Set aside to cool and drain on paper towels.
2. Drain all but 1 tbsp of bacon grease from skillet. Add spinach and cook over medium high heat until completely wilted and cooked through. Sprinkle spinach with salt and set aside on butting board to cool.
3. Add onion to skillet and cook until translucent and a tiny bit golden at the edges.
4. Add garlic to onion in skillet and cook for 1 minute. Remove from heat.
5. Place cream cheese in large bowl. Stir in shredded cheese, onions and garlic.
6. Chop cooked spinach into very fine bits and stir into cheese mixture.
7. Chop cooked bacon into very fine bits and stir HALF into cheese mixture. Set the other half of bacon aside.
8. Stir cayenne pepper into cheese mixture.
9. Combine walnuts and remaining bacon on a plate or shallow dish.
10. Roll the cream cheese mixture into teaspoon-sized balls, then roll each ball into nuts and bacon bits.
11. Wrap tightly and refrigerate until serving.

NOTE: You can make one big cheese ball rather than small ones.

BEAN SALAD:

This is my own creation and it works well with many entrees and side dishes.

Ingredients:
1 can green beans
1 can yellow beans
1 can kidney beans
1 cup lima beans

I add any or all of the following:

1 bell pepper (choose your colour)
celery
onion (I like purple ones)

Kraft Classic Herb salad dressing OR Italian salad dressing
sweetner

Instructions:

1. Drain the beans.
2. Mix all ingredients together with the salad dressing.
3. Sweeten to taste using sweetner.
4. Marinate in refrigerator.

1 serving = 1 cup = 6 carbs

Bacon and Onion Green Beans:
(from lowcarblayla.blogspot.ca)

Ingredients:

3 slice bacon
1/2 onion, diced
1 tbsp Worcestershire sauce (optional)
1/2 pound green beans, frozen or fresh, but not canned
salt and pepper to taste

Instructions:

1. Cut the bacon into small pieces. Chop onion. Cook bacon and onion together in small skillet over medium heat, stirring occasionally.
2. Wash beans, if using fresh. Put in microwave safe bowl with 1 tbsp water. Microwave 3 to 4 minutes.
3. Once bacon looks close to done, add green beans, worcestershire, salt and pepper to skillet. Stir occasionally. Cook until beans soften (may have to add another tbsp of water while cooking, if beans seem to be drying up.)

Makes 4 servings. 1 serving = 4.5 carbs

DESSERTS AND OTHER TREATS

For diabetics, the topic of dessert, and specifically sugar, is usually a loaded conversation, but through experience, I have found that deprivation is the mother of failure. If I feel deprived of some of the wonderful treats in life, my mindset becomes stuck in a negative place and invariably I feel like "cheating" to make myself feel better. My challenge became, how can I enjoy a "sweet treat" without affecting my blood sugar and gaining weight? Luckily, the internet provided a whole world of delicious answers. Here are some of my favourite recipes that help us enjoy our food without jeopardizing our health.

CRUSTLESS PUMPKIN PIE:
(from justapinch.com)

This one's a winner! You would think you were eating regular pumpkin pie! Thanksgiving dinner with the family is a great time to try this one out on non-diabetics. They won't believe how authentic and light this tastes!

Ingredients:

1 can pumpkin (15 oz.)
1 can evaporated milk (12 oz.)
3 egg whites
1/2 tsp salt
1 tbsp pumpkin pie spice
1 tbsp cinnamon
1 tsp vanilla
2/3 cups Splenda

Instructions:

1. Combine all ingredients until smooth and pour into pie plate.
2. Bake at 400 F. for 15 minutes, then 325 F. for 45 minutes.
3. Top with dollop of low-fat whipped topping, cut into 8 slices.

1 slice = 69 calories, 6 carbs

OAT MUFFINS:
(This is my own recipe. My dietitian helped me tweak it to reduce the carb content without affecting the taste or texture.)

Ingredients:

1 cup oats
1 cup buttermilk
1 cup flour
1 tsp baking powder
1/2 tsp baking soda
1/2 tsp salt
1/2 cup Stevia (or other sweetner)
1/4 cup brown sugar
1 egg
1/4 cup melted margarine
1 cup blueberries, cranberries, raisins or chocolate chips (or 1/2 cup blueberries and 1/2 cup cranberries)

Instructions:

1. Combine all ingredients and pour into muffin cups.
2. Bake at 375F. for 20 to 25 minutes.

1 muffin = 15 carbs

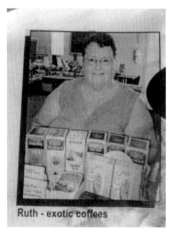

Me at my heaviest
2009

CHOCOLATE CHEESECAKE CUPCAKES:
(from culinarytuesdays.com)

This is one delicious treat! My friends raved about this, and you will too!

Ingredients:

1 box Devil's Food cake mix
6 oz. container of Chobani 0% plain Greek yogurt
1 tsp vanilla
1 egg
1 cup water

(for the cheesecake)
3 oz. reduced fat cream cheese
1/4 cup Chobani 0% vanilla Greek yogurt
1/4 reduced fat sour cream
2 large egg whites
1/4 cup sugar
1 tsp vanilla

Instructions:

1. Preheat oven to 350 F.
2. Prepare 22 cupcake tins with paper liners.
3. In a medium mixing bowl, beat all the cheesecake ingredients until well combined, set aside.
4. In a large mixing bowl, beat all the cake ingredients until well combined.
5. Add chocolate cake mixture to the paper liners approx. 1/2 full.
6. Add a small ice cream scoop of the cheesecake mixture on top of the cake mixture.
7. Repeat for all 22 cupcakes.
8. Swirl with a fork to combine the cheesecake and the cake at the top.
9. Bake for 30 mins.
10. Cool and store in fridge for at least 1 hour before serving.

1 cupcake = 137 calories, 19 carbs, .5g fibre

CREAM PUFFS:
(from kraftcanada.com)

This recipe is carb and calorie friendly, and makes an absolutely divine dessert for company! Try it and you'll see what I mean!

Ingredients:

1/2 cup water
2 tbsp. butter
1/2 cup flour
2 eggs
1 pkg. (4 serving size) Jello Vanilla Fat Free Instant Pudding
1 cup cold skim milk
3/4 cup thawed Cool Whip Light Whipped Topping
1 oz. Baker's dark chocolate

Instructions:

1. Heat oven to 400 F.
2. Bring water and butter to boil in large saucepan. Add flour. Remove from heat. Stir vigourously until well blended. Return to heat; cook and stir on medium heat 2 mins. or until mixture pulls away from side of pan and forms a ball. Cool 5 mins. Add eggs, one at a time, beating with wooden spoon after each until well blended. Drop 2 inches apart, into 16 small mounds on baking sheets sprayed with cooking spray.
3. Bake 25 mins. until golden brown. Remove to wire racks; cool completely. Meanwhile beat pudding mix and milk in medium bowl with whisk 2 mins. Stir in Cool Whip. Refrigerate until ready to use.
4. Cut puffs horizontally in half with serrated knife, remove any soft dough from inside puffs. Fill bottoms of puffs with pudding mixutre; replace tops. Melt chocolate as directed on package; drizzle over cream puffs. Keep refrigerated.

1 puff = 35 calories, 4g carbs

YOGURT BARK - LOW CARB:
(from Andres Regalado at the-lowcarb-diet.com: I found this recipe on Pinterest)

Try this for a tasty snack! You will feel like you're eating candy!

Ingredients:

2 cups plain yogurt
1/2 cup sweetner
2 medium strawberries, chopped
2 tbsp pistachios

Instructions:

1. Mix sweetener and yogurt together. Pour into freezer proof dish.
2. Top yogurt with strawberries and pistachios.
3. Freeze for 3 hours or until bark is solid. Remove from freezer and let sit for 5 minutes. Break into 12 pieces.
4. Serve immediately or store in freezer safe bags for one month.

1 piece = 42 calories, 5.67 carbs

"JUST ONE" OATMEAL COOKIE
(from eatingwelllivingthin -- I found this one on Pinterest too!)

Who doesn't love an oatmeal cookie with a cup of your favourite hot beverage on a cold day? This one's a winner!

Ingredients:

1 tsp melted butter
1 1/2 tsp Egg Beaters or whipped regular egg
1 1/2 tbsp oatmeal, old-fashioned or quick
2 tsp Splenda Granular (I used Stevia and would recommend a little less)
pinch of salt
pinch of cinnamon
drop of vanilla

Instructions:

Mix all ingredients well and drop on a cookie sheet. Flatten slightly. Bake at 350F for 8-10 minutes. Makes 9 cookies.

1 cookie = 69 calories, 3 g net carbs

TO MAKE A LARGER BATCH, use:

1/3 cup melted butter
1/8 tsp salt
1/8 tsp baking powder
1 egg OR 1/4 cup Egg Beaters
2/3 cup Splenda Granular
1 tsp vanilla
1/8 tsp cinnamon
1 1/3 cup oatmeal

"Love yourself enough to live a healthy lifestyle." -Author Unknown

PEANUT PECAN COOKIES:
(from Company's Coming - Low Carb, by Jean Pare)

This is an excellent recipe by an excellent cook! Jean Pare says these are "crunchy, delicate cookies." I experimented with this one by using 1/4 cup Stevia and 1/4 cup brown sugar. I also added 1 tbsp of cocoa for a different taste. Increase the pecans to 1/2 cup for a nuttier flavour.

Ingredients:

1/2 cup brown sugar, packed
1/4 tsp baking powder
1 cup crunchy peanut butter
1 large egg
1/4 cup finely chopped pecans

Instructions:

1. Combine brown sugar and baking powder in medium bowl. Add peanut butter. Beat until smooth. Add egg. Beat well.
2. Add pecans. Stir. Roll dough into 1 inch balls. Arrange balls about 1 1/2 inches apart, on ungreased cookie sheets. Flatten with fork.
3. Bake at 325F for about 8 minutes until tops are set. Let stand on cookie sheets for 5 minutes before removing to wire racks to cool. Makes 36 cookies.

1 cookie = 65 calories, 5 g. carbs, 1 g. fibre

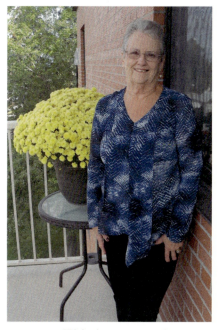

This is me now!
September 2015

ACKNOWLEDGEMENTS

My sincere and deepest thanks go out to all of the people who assisted and supported me in this project -- both in helping me to become a healthier person, and in compiling this booklet.

The professional staff at the Diabetes Clinic at Norfolk General Hospital in Simcoe, Ontario, deserve my deepest appreciation for helping me change my life. Most specifically, I'd like to acknowledge the friendship and support of my dietitian, Jessica Brown, who made it a pleasure to check in each month. Her warm and compassionate attitude towards me was the catalyst I needed to lose weight and control my blood sugar. She is one in a million.

To my friends, Jean Mottashed, who put my thoughts into words, and George Mottashed for technical assistance, I appreciate your diligent attention to this project. To Caitlin and Brad Mottashed, for editing, formatting and creating the cover, my sincere thanks. I never thought something like this would be possible. Together you all made my dreams come true.

To Jen and Colin Barber my heartfelt thanks for their unconditional support and affection. They were my "taste-testers" when I experimented with different recipes and my cheerleaders when I needed a cheering section.

And to my grand-daughters, Brittney, Mackenzie and Cailyn, for their precious love. These girls are the reason I hope to live a long, happy and healthy life.

Made in the USA
Middletown, DE
17 January 2019